Table of Contents

Page

Light up hope with life energy

We do our daily routine by not taking into account many things in life. The state of dullness that comes out of our comfort zone generates life energy but when there is a widespread crisis that wakes you up from sleep, you suddenly realize the uncertainty of life. Now you come out of your comfort zone, then you are forced to find new ways to handle yourself. People should learn from this crisis that If life is not eternal, then the facilities and problems in life will not always be there. Light up hope with life energy

Spirituality is helpful in a crisis

Being depressed in crisis and problems means that you are lacking in spirituality. Depression causes suicidal tendencies, so the reason is that whenever you are in a low level of energy, you cannot see outside your small world that you have created, you only see your distress, your eyes are closed even after opening. When you open your eyes then you will see that many people are in crisis. Prayer meditation, yoga, and pranayama help a person to see beyond his limits and create education to face challenges.

The crisis also awakens human values in you. In the last few months, when India along with the world has been badly affected by the Corona virus, then people of all religions came forward to help each other, a sense of recognition increased. Then we all realized that there is a lot of love and oneness in the world.

Service is the source of joy

The source of joy in service is that people who serve do their best in bad times. When there is a disaster or a war, then volunteers of humanitarian institutions remain calm and stable because they are immersed in service. The more comfort they give to people, the more they feel happy. On the other hand, the selfish people who want to enjoy themselves only remain unhappy even in good times. Often in good times, people lose their happiness on some small thing. A wise man is happy even in bad times. An ignorant person remains unhappy even in good times. Time is not good or bad. You make time good or bad. Generally, people blame bad times and then wait for the good times. But even if an astrologer claims that your time is going bad, only then it is you who can make your time good.

Save devotion and Faith

The good or the bad time has an effect on you, but also know that you are more than time and you can pass efficiently from that time because of your absolute relationship with God. Give importance to human and spiritual values, because in times of crisis, reverence goes on and in times of distress, trust goes away.

There is a story of a newly married couple of Japan. They were going on a honeymoon in the village and suddenly a storm came. The woman was terrified but the man was in peace and always smiling, then the woman asked the husband " I am nervous and frightened that this boat will sink, but you are smiling, we can die by drowning". Suddenly the husband took his knife and put it on the wife's neck, the woman started laughing and said this is not the time to joke. Think about the future. The husband said why are you not afraid of me that I will kill you. The wife started laughing. What do I need to worry about? I believe that you will not harm me but instead will protect me from that knife. The husband replied that I have the same relationship with nature and God. My life is in the hands of God, so he will not let me die in this storm, so the door of my life is in his hand, so why do I need to worry about it. At that moment the wife started praying with her husband. Within few moments the storm got stopped. The moral of the story is that in crisis when faith should be required it disappears. Devotion is a gift from God, we should believe in God

The present is the key to a happy future

The moment in our hands is the present, the future we don't know the past that has gone. Present continues continuously, is under our control, yet no such provision has been developed that we can correct our old mistakes by entering the pastor enter the future and make it beautiful and return to the present. So why do we cry about the past or worry about the future?

Because our future depends on the activities of the past, so if we develop our present before it becomes past, then surely the future will be good. To change life for the better requires actionable things in the present. The present may be very important for us so that we can invest in improving our unseen future. It was said that in the refuge of love there is no past and future. It is very important to live in the present to love life.

Let us make use of every moment, we should spend every moment of our work in human welfare, the people who put their work on tomorrow do not respect their present and later they have to regret that the famous painter Rizwan used to say that I am making this right now, this is my best painting, this notion picks up the person, whether we make pictures written in poetry or do any work, our effort is to do the best for the present work.

The effect of the past is that it tries to tie in its magic. If an artist considers some creativity in the past to be his best, then his creativity gets the same end. All the work that has been done in the past, the best will be the work going on in the present. We should not stick to the past but learn from the mistakes of the past.

The past is the laboratory of the future. By learning from the mistakes of the past; the present is the stage of deep thinking. Some people also affect their future by past mistakes. The past should remain a team of learning only. Successful humans learn from the past and move towards success. And they have a keen eye on the present planet.

Understanding Mindfulness and its benefits

Mindfulness is the ability to be fully present at the moment. Understanding Mindfulness and its benefits are really important for us. Thinking about the past, future, or any other event that takes us away from the present is not mindfulness. Being present at the moment involves us being aware of where we are. What are we doing, and how are we feeling. And more, it is being aware of ourselves, knowing our limits, and understanding our goals and desires in life.

As humans, it is easy to get carried away by other thoughts events, and certain circumstances This causes adverse effects on our brain, on our physical, mental, and emotional health. For example, stress at the Workplace can distract us from appreciating our family, which can cause problems at home and family. Mindfulness can help at that cause.

All people are mentally capable, even if it seems hard. Our brains are fully capable of focusing on the present and honoring the outside deflections of life. That being said, it can be incredibly difficult to do so. This is the reason why mindfulness practice is so helpful. Mindfulness can teach us and train us to focus better on the present, allowing us to ignore anything else that can be a distraction.

Understanding the point of mindfulness

Before starting your mindfulness journey, it is important to understand what Mindfulness can't do for you. If you have unrealistic expectations regarding Mindfulness, it can be easy to realize that Mindfulness is not working and giving up on practice altogether.

Many people believe that the state of mind is about attaining some state of bliss. Ananda or Bliss is often described as some state of absolute happiness that is forgotten for other factors surrounding this. It is important to recognize that mindfulness, is not about reaching a state of bliss. It is impossible to reach this state because there are always challenges and difficulties in life that act as a hindrance to attain a state of bliss or a so-called state. In other words, bliss does not exist to say for a normal human facing life challenges.

That being said, mindfulness can and should make you feel happy and more content with your overall life, but it's more realistic about it. This allows attention to appreciate your life and yourself better. It helps you see past short-term conflicts and appreciate life. You have it even faced in bad times.

For this reason, the act of mindfulness helps you live a better life. Living your life involves more content in your situation, responding with more compassion and rationally in difficult situations, more realistic, love with yourself and others. Is not about creating a perfect life, but it's about creating the life you want and excited to live with always.

If you think it's a matter of mind, you can say it more easily. Set realistic goals for your mindfulness training. These goals should reflect your present abilities and your future that you are actively pursuing yourself to live the Ideal Life you want to.

It is important to note that mindfulness is not about being in the present time. As human beings, we will be completely overwhelmed. We currently stayed all day, every day, if overloaded. There are times when in our life we should not think of the past, future, or anything.

Benefits of mindfulness

The effects of mindfulness have been studied by several clinical trials, allowing us to believe that mindfulness improves our overall health and wellbeing. For example, mindfulness can improve the following conditions:

- Stress

- Worry

- Pain

- Depression

- Blood pressure

- Insomnia

- Diabetes

- Cardiovascular disease

Mindfulness also helps to increase attention, control emotions, and increase motivation and overall life satisfaction. Together, these advantages allow you to experience a healthy and happy life.

Mindfulness is the act of being in the present so that you can live one healthy and happy life. As you become more mindful, you will experience many benefits in your emotional, mental, and physical health.

There is no better time than being at present. Keep your health in mind and make it a priority. To get started, start small, include mindfulness in your daily routine, setting a time in the day for a long mindful practice, try new things, and be kind to yourself.

Although it can be difficult to get caught up in the groove of mindfulness at first, you will quickly understand that being mindful is a total asset to your overall well-being and life. No matter whether you are on your own mindful or life journey, be kind and patient with yourself. If you do not talk to yourself in a way that is respectful and kind, then there is no way to truly live in your mind and appreciate your life. Kindness is the main takeaway of this article. If you don't learn anything else, learn to treat yourself the way you would treat your best friend.

Meditation - Find freedom from Attachments

With the help of Meditation, we can find freedom from all type of worldly Attachments that act as a hindrance in our mental and spiritual well being.

In our practical life the things that are useful or purposeful for us, only the inner conscious can find the right answer to it. Eating, drinking, and living in peace is all for the fulfillment of our mental well being. Important thing is that reasoning or logical thinking is related to our Consciousness. So it is to be justified that spiritualism can be attained relating to a human's Conscious level of his sense of mindfulness.

By regular practice of Sadhna or meditation, a human being can find his true path of spiritual enlightenment. The pure state of bliss is one such philosophy. By following spiritual practices we will find the true state of blessedness or pure happiness that is permanent and absolute and cannot be found with any other means but only with the way of following spiritual practices.

According to our Conscious level, we can find real knowledge of destruction or development. With the increase in the level of our Consciousness, we start to find happiness, beginning from a small segment or section to a holistic level of inner joy that we call the state of blessedness. In this process, we start to find happiness and give preference to deep mental peace rather than any physical pleasure of desires and attachments. We tend to leave these pleasures aside.

Attachments and desires cause attraction that diverts our attention and acts as a hindrance to our spiritual growth. These desires give birth to a new desire for the completion of previous desires.

For Country's love or any such rare happiness, a human does not fear to surrender or give his life for it. There are thousands of such examples in history. This is a human's higher level of Consciousness or a healthy mindset.

By the practice of Ashtanga Yoga, a devotee or practitioner can slowly and steadily grow his thinking power and with that developed thinking, he can find spiritual awakening. By this spiritual awakening, he can find true happiness. We should know that without natural knowledge it is not possible to do so. We should increase to raise allegiance or fidelity. By inclination only, allegiance will rise and with the growth of the allegiance, we will be blessed by god's Grace.

With only a little of God's Grace, we find freedom from attachment with this physical structure or body. Perpetual perversion discretion is awakened and this discretion develops us to Brahmroop or immortal. It is to be noted that In the meditation route the biggest thing is devotion or allegiance.

How to begin the practice of meditation

Sit down with leg crossed, back straight, and eyes closed. Beware of your breath around the nostrils, as you breathe in and as you breathe out. Breathe in, experiencing the whole body, breathe out, experiencing the whole body. Breathe in, relaxing the whole body, breathe out, relaxing the whole body. Always mindful, breathe in, mindful, breathe out. Open your eyes and come out of meditation.

How to begin your practice ?

Begin with a short period of 10-15 minutes. Slowly increase the duration. One hour is a good span for daily meditation.

Benefits

• Sooths and calms the mind

• Relieves tension and anxiety

• Helps to reduce high blood pressure

• Effective for insomnia

• Improves concentration

• Builds self-confidence

Keeping in line with meditation can greatly increase the effectiveness of the process, as you can not only learn to perform better but also strengthen your mind's ability to concentrate and calm down.

When you can experience the positive benefits of meditation, a repeated practice not only helps keep your mind calm for longer but also enables you to gain a greater degree of mental clarity and well being.

Yoga Conscience - Moral rationality of the Soul

Yoga is an art. A way of living. It originates from our Conscience that heals our body mind and soul spiritually. We can say that yoga is the food of the Soul. The food or diet we consume for our daily physical activities but for the soul, the food is the yoga that involves breathing, asanas, meditation, several kriyas with proper discipline.

It is a proven fact that the roots of yoga are inherited in our Conscience. The will or resolute should be to motivate self to grow the roots continuously in an unconscious manner and to transform the roots into a huge tree that that will flower our life so that it may be fruitful to all of us. Life will be blissful and prosperous in wisdom.

Conscience is the moral rationality of the soul. Yoga is the action process derived from our Conscience where it is deep-rooted. Then it becomes a natural phenomenon of action in everything we do and perform. This routine is similar to our breathing system that happens subconsciously without putting any effort.

This is the Conscience that heals us in a subconscious way that motivates us constantly in our every action that makes us believe that missing yoga sometimes makes us uneasy and interference in gaining divine energy.

Yoga Conscience is the art of liberation from our desires and constantly grow our energy level. It is the belief in our moral values. The increased level in our self-confidence. It makes us strong. The inherent belief that we can overcome all obstacles and hindrance in whatever we face or get surrounded with. The hope of no illness, healthy, and fit. The increase of immunity and will to win. The growth in our energy level.

Conscience and life are interrelated deeply. A newborn baby shows a glimpse of his presence in one or the other way. For adults, conscience takes birth in another form. He acts according to the situation. Conscience is itself a form of awakening unknowingly or reaction according to situation and surroundings.

If we look at history we will find so many great people that have left their signs of greatness facing and fighting immense obstacles and problems but they have never left the fire of their Conscience. These great people were not only their country ideals but the light bearer for the entire society and mankind.

The belief cannot be negated that the Conscience general basics are connected to Indian mythology and the Vedas. We can thus understand the Conscience in Vedic, Dharma, or religious, the cultural concept only. Yoga is born from this concept of Conscience.

When in our daily routines we see or hear any inhuman act, our state of mind screams. We feel frustrated, pathetic, and agonized. Any indifference or such a sinful act by the evildoer means his senses are lost. He cannot differentiate between right or wrong. His Conscience is dead.

Actually, in our lifespan, we define good or the bad to the level of our Conscience. This is our Conscience we develop the thinking process or mechanics that gives birth to wishes and feelings. Often feelings subdue our thinking process. Knowingly in control of wishes, we are trapped in our feelings and then we try to escape from right thinking. To not to face this, we should always try to scratch the right Conscience. Spiritual knowledge is effective in this scenario. Although it is possible only by awakening of our Conscience.

Yoga Conscience is beyond our minds. While the mind behaves rationally for our decision process or thought process but Conscience is the self-guidance of rightness or wrongness of the thought process. The awareness of our action to do right.

So Yoga should not be confined to just poses and exercises alone but the Conscience is the motivation of its holistic benefits to our overall well being and not only to gain physical benefits but also spiritual awakening to become a liberated soul. Yoga Conscience is the effort of fulfillment that we always struggled to live in peace, to live in silence, to be within ourselves, to discover our trueness, and be our own masters.

The law of energy flow in yoga

Energy is eternal and all around that grows within us when we arouse it by following yoga practices. There is an energy yoga routine we should know. Yoga ignites this energy that is divine and blissful that surrounds us or grasps us internally and externally. The source of this energy is a regular flow of prana yoga within us. This is the energy we are searching for that is flowing freely and vibrantly by doing yoga practices energy or boosting yoga exercises that involve breathing, asanas, meditation. This we can call us energy flow yoga sequence. Self-awareness, discipline, and right guidance is strictly observed in all these yoga practices that become a habit in all our actions and deeds that we do.

What is that energy that grows slowly and steadily that we feel and are regularly motivated to grow that blissful energy? What is the concept of energy in yoga ? Yes, certainly there is a law of energy a yogi should know and feel and practice to gain or grow that eternal energy slowly and steadily that is the very base of yoga. We can say it as the root of yoga. The energy flow yoga sequence. Physical exercise, asanas, mudras are all subsidiary to gain real resource or energy.

Energy flow yoga sequence

Food – Energy gain

Sleep – Energy maintained / Stored

Awakening – Energy released

Pranayama – Energy is Awakened

Pledge / Dhaarna – Energy is focused

Meditation / Dhyan – Movement of energy upwards

Fear – Energy shrinks

Desire – Movement of energy downwards

Love- Flow of energy everywhere that is elaborate and extensive

Samadhi – Energy combines with the divine being. Merge with the universe.

Let us discuss the above factors in detail

Food – The food or diet that we intake daily to perform our daily activities is the source of energy we gain. The food should be sattvic and pure. Sattvic food removes toxins from our body and prevents us from many ailments.

Sleep – A good sleep makes us afresh and energetic. Energy is maintained or restored in the cycle of sleep. Sleeping time frame should make us relax and energetic to perform our daily activities. Sleep disorders cause various problems and depletion of energy level that is negative for energy growth.

Awakening – Awakening is a process of regular growing, knowing us inherently, to conquer desires and limitations, rising above senses. It is a continuous process of being on our horizon to be awake in all our minute activities. A process of vigils and alertness to our divine existence. In the process of awakening, energy is released.

Pranayama – Pranayama or breathing is very beneficial to us. In this state, the energy is awakened or aroused. Pranayama should be done regularly. Morning time is the best for that. Anulom vilom or alternate nostril breathing should be done with the same preference as breathing. Breathing regenerates our cells thus healing the body.

Dharana / Pledge – This is the state when energy is focused due to concentration and cultivation of inner sensory activities or awareness.

Dhyan / Meditation – Dhyan or meditation on the divine is an ultimate source of energy moving upwards. This is the state of bliss.

Fear – Yoga practitioners should not fear from unknown. Yoga practices remove fear and anxiety. Energy shrinks here.

Desire – Our desires prone us to worldly pleasures and attractions that cause diverting our attention to unwanted things and unnecessary needs. This consumes our lot of energy. This results in the movement of energy downwards. We should practice to control or limit our desires that always grows with each desire fulfilled and becomes a never-ending process.

Love – Love is a universal divine phenomenon that bounds us to nature and mankind. It is a sense of responsibility and devotion to each creature created by the supreme. Here flow of energy is elaborate and extensive thus healing self and society.

Samadhi – Samadhi is the ultimate stage of energy flow that combines with the divine being and merge with the universe.

We have discussed the law of flow of energy in yoga which every yogi or yoga practitioner should know and understand and try to aim to gain that energy levels before following the yoga journey.

Yogic way to Stay fit while at work

A consistent fitness routine is the best way to keep your body in good physical shape and your mind healthy. There is a yogic way to stay fit while at work. Being active does not mean that you need to spend many hours in the gym. Doing the things you love, such as walking in the rain, swimming and spending time with loved ones in the forest is the best way to exercise. You can also find ways to fit in some essential work activities, such as taking the stairs and getting up from your desk to walk a short distance every hour.

A typical employee sits in front of his desk for eight hours or more, answering telephone calls, surfing the Internet, writing office communications, and other desk-bound tasks. Sitting all day increases the likelihood of obesity. There are risks of having poor posture, muscle cramps, and backache. Stretching and deep breathing techniques on your desk can help keep you free from pain and stress during work.

Stretching is an important and easy way to reduce back pain and neck strain. Maintain a flat posture by adjusting the height of your chair and placing your spine behind your chair. This will keep your back and neck bulging and less likely to turn forward which will cause cramps and headaches.

To activate your chest and shoulders during a long day at work, plunge the chair. Place both hands on the arms of your chair and slowly raise your arms down while straightening your arms. Take yourself back down and stop when your floor is a few inches from the seat, count 5. 15 times. Avoid both wrists by turning both your wrists in circles 10 times.

For lower body stiffness, try to stretch your lower leg alternately, right and left. Then, sitting in your chair, raise one leg and straighten it, but do not bend your knees, count to three and keep your leg down and hold for several seconds. Do this again with your other leg.

More calories are burned than standing and sitting. Instead of using the phone to talk with your colleagues, go to their desk and talk face to face. Stand and stretch your body to answer phone calls. This will give your body a little rest and will also build a stronger relationship with your colleagues.

Bike for walking or working. If you ride a bus or metro, get off at a few blocks or earlier stops and walk the rest of the way. Walking ten extra minutes a day can help you burn extra calories and make you feel more vibrant. Climb stairs instead of lifts for stepping towards your fitness goals. Use a pedometer to monitor your physical activity and reminds you to keep going. A pedometer is a small device that counts every step you take.

Bringing in fitness gear will also help. Bring a yoga mat that you can use during your break, or a stretch ball to relax your hands and fingers after using the computer. You can also do push-ups while waiting. Resistance bands – Stretch cords or tubes that offer weight-like resistance when you pull over them – curl some hands on cabinets or drawers and between functions.

Organize groups running lunchtime with your teammates. Encourage everyone to get regular exercise at work and even at home. Schedule walking meetings, if the weather cooperates, take out your walking meetings. Having regularly scheduled exercise time with your team is a great way to ensure that you exercise on a consistent basis and will build friendships in a shared activity that you can enjoy weekly.

Keep an eye on your diet, eating habits and food intake. This is the most important thing. No one can exercise for a poor diet. Eating cooked vegetables will give you nutrition and improve your digestion. A homemade lunch instead of vending machine goodies will save your wallet and trim your waistline. Drink warm water before, during and after your activities to stay hydrated. Every system in your body needs water to avoid energy drain and fatigue.

Avoid long hours in front of the TV at home. Your eyes must be tired due to work on computer and screen. Give your eyes a rest. And fall asleep before 10:00 at night. Resting tomorrow and saving more energy for tomorrow. You may also be able to get up and work before work!

Being active is not difficult. Just keep your body moving. Track your progress and make it easy and fun. You will keep your body fit and also build strong relationships with the people around you. And it will lead you to a life full of joy!

How to integrate yoga into a work

It can be a challenge to fulfill all your activities and obligations, even on ordinary days. When you have various professional and personal responsibilities to attend, you may struggle to fit into everything. As anxiety increases, it is common to lose your peace. Restore your balance and take care of yourself by incorporating some yoga in your daily work routine.

Be Conscious

An important aspect of yoga involves mindfulness. When you focus on stress and what triggers it, you can help reduce it. For example, if a colleague tries to press your button, what can you do to avoid an interchange with this person. When you have no choice, center yourself and work on regaining your inner peace. Even concentrating on breathing for just a short period of time can be effective for slowing a racing heart and refreshing an anxious mind.

Desk exercise

Many yoga poses are ideal while you sit at the desk. These actions are not comprehensive or difficult, and if you work in an office with others, they will not draw attention to you.

– Pranayama will help you to center yourself when tension increases. Sit in your chair and focus on connecting from your feet. Position your chin so that it is parallel to the floor and center your shoulders on your hips. Start breathing calmly while inhaling your breath. Stop for few seconds and exhale the breath. Repeat the process from five to ten times.

– Sit on the edge of your seat, and place your feet on the floor. Keep your fingers behind your back. Inhale deeply, move your hands towards the floor and chest upward. Hold your breath for a few seconds and then exhale completely. Again repeat the process
Standing exercise

– Standing straight and bend at the hips to touch your toes. Holding this simple pose for a few seconds is often effective for fighting stress and calming the brain.
– Keep your hands behind your hips, directly behind your back. Raise your crossed hands as high as possible. When lifting, focus on lifting your sternum. Hold the lift for at least 30 seconds, and then let it go. Repeat this movement several times.

Even if you cannot step and spread on the floor, the way you practice yoga, you can get some benefit from doing these movements throughout the day. In many cases, colleagues will not even realize what you are doing when you stretch and soothe the pain to breathe.

Yoga helping us in hard times or bad days

These are the days of Corona. How yoga helping us in hard times of Corona. Sometimes it happens that everything seems to be going wrong in our lives. Everything seems to be deteriorating and our efforts to stop it from worsening more or reversing for good is not happening. We are currently experiencing it and you may also experience it. I am lucky to have friends and family members who love me and are always ready to help me in my time of need but I like to practice yoga before I go to someone else's help because it is often at such a time, my situation changes.

Given below are 4 ways yoga that helps us in bad times:

Getting out of our discomfort. Letting go of despair or hope is never going to change the situation. Many times it has happened to us that we felt as if we are going to fall while in the position of the warrior. However, when we stopped thinking about it and started taking deep breaths while calming our mind we are able to balance for longer. This useful lesson that we learned by doing yoga can be applied to other parts of life as well.

Remind us that we are stronger than we think. At first, when we saw someone doing arm balances, we imagined how strong that person is. We simply made the assumption that we could never do this. However, when we started looking deeper into our body, we are able to do it within a month enabling strengthening our body and understanding our strength level in our body!.We increase our odds by thinking that we cannot handle them. We must always remember that we are stronger than we think. Whenever we suffer from bad times, we remember the first time we are able to balance completely.

Increases our focus on the positive. Yoga practice helps me realize the positive around us. Too much negativity also spoils our scenario in all cases. It tells us that life does not matter, I am lucky that I am alive and my breath is still coming in and going out. It gives us great comfort.

Reminds that everything is temporary. This is a very useful lesson that helps reduce the negativity inside us. Of course, everything in this world is temporary – from pain in happiness to bad times of happiness. Life goes on no matter what happens. Therefore, instead of remembering the beauty of the present time, we will do nothing by paying attention to how good everything will be. Do not miss it!

5 Poses that can help us At the End of A Bad Day

Usually during any bad day we would come home, eat some snacks while drinking coffee and watch a romantic comedy to get us ready to cook dinner. For a few hours, our attention was towards something else. All these things give us temporary happiness that was necessary to do something else because as you would already know, the end of a bad day breaks us down in such a way that we don't like to do anything at that time. But after all these things were over, we felt tired and lethargic – thus preparing ourselves for another bad day. In fact, when we spend more time avoiding our bad day than we live, we actually face a lot of problems.

We should know that to prevent this from happening, some changes had to be made to our routine, so we have to change the schedule and to do yoga everyday if we are not doing it. We should decide to do yoga at any cost and to give some time to it.

Below are some of the poses we can do and say that they are life saving at the end of a bad day. You can also try them and feel the difference yourself:

Child Pose: This is one of the best poses to find happiness. When you take a deep breath and melt on the floor in a baby pose, you take care of yourself and allow your body to listen to your intuition.

Viprita Karani: This is a restorative pose. You can try it on a bolt or on top of a blanket. This greatly reduces the amount of stress and helps in simulation. Only five minutes can make a difference for the whole day.

Downward-Facing Dog Pose: We don't like going to any yoga class, which doesn't include a downward-facing dog in any way. This posture helps a lot in getting maximum relief when you feel stressed. To do this easily we can place our head either on a bolt or on top of a blanket.

Shoulderstand: This can be difficult for many of you, but just one minute of this pose can go a long way in getting the bad thoughts out of your mind.

Savasna: This posture is also one of the best for relaxing the tired brain. It is a posture in which you simply relax, breathe and absorb the benefits of your yoga practice.

Living a healthy life

Everyone wants to live happy and healthy living. This can be done by practice of yoga daily or every day. Yoga is a popular form of exercise that has been known to mankind for more than 5,000 years. Yoga is a traditional method of meditation; developed in ancient times in India. Most people are aware of the fact that yoga and meditation can help anyone to have some great health benefits.

It is one of the most effective and successful therapy that keep the human body and mind healthy. On a physical level, yoga relieves from many diseases. Practicing different postures gives strength to your body and makes you mentally and physically fit.

Yoga can soak your mind and body properly. If you want to know how Yoga can help you heal yourself, then you need to read the article below carefully. To heal your body you must first start loving yourself.

Now we are going to discuss in detail about how Yoga can help you to heal properly. Make sure you look at the points below carefully.

• Yoga helps you to keep your mind absolutely relaxed and calm. If you want to be relaxed all the time, then yoga can definitely help you a lot. You got to make sure that you make the right choice every time. You should give your body some extra time to heal. You can start by practicing some simple yoga moves and asanas. How can you bring it to the groove?

• The power of acceptance is the strongest ever. You can really benefit a lot from it. You just have to accept your mistakes and strengths as they are. It is useless to be sad at anything. Well, you just have to accept the reality and move on. You can put all your efforts and energy into learning yoga. Tell your trainer about any issues that are bothering you.

• Healing is all about being happy. If you are looking for some enjoyment then you need to practice yoga regularly. You can do anything that makes you happy. You can incorporate yoga into your regular lifestyle. If you are looking for something more fun, you can consider practicing it with your loved ones.

• If you want to take good care of your health then practice caution and mantras. Yoga can help you to cure many disorders including back pain and abdominal pain. You just have to follow the right fitness regime and exercise right.

• The art of letting things go is one of the hardest to learn. It is often said that a person who learns to let things go easily is happiest. So, yoga helps you in this. Regular practice allows you to be healthy easily under all circumstances. You can also learn how to be patient in the most difficult situations.

These are some of the most important things that you should remember about practicing yoga. You need to make sure that if you want to heal your body completely, then you do some yoga yoga regularly. If you are looking for some more information then you can surf the internet. Have lots of fun and have lots of fun.

Today, due to its many benefits, Yoga is one of the leading names in the healthcare and wellness industry, which is why it is important for you to know some more benefits in detail.

Flexibility

Yoga involves the movement and stretch of body parts in many ways. Therefore, it increases flexibility. After a certain period of time, you will be able to gain flexibility in your back, hips and shoulders. However, with age, flexibility naturally decreases which further leads to immobility and pain. Yoga has the ability to modify and postpone this process.

Power

There are many yoga postures that help in weight loss in various ways. The body becomes stronger by giving different poses for a certain period of time.

Muscle tone

Muscle toning is a by-product of yoga. As your body gets stronger, muscle toning increases. Yoga also shapes lean and long muscles.

The balance

A position like standing on one leg helps improve balance. This is one of the most important benefits of doing yoga as we move towards old age.

Pain Relieve

Strength and enhanced flexibility helps in the prevention of back pain, legs or any other part of the body. Nowadays many people complain of back pain due to long working hours on computer. It can also give rise to spinal compression. In such cases, yoga is one of the best treatments without any side effects. It helps in preventing any type of body pain.

Better breathing

Stress is one of the main reasons behind breathing problems. Pranayama is an exercise in yoga that satisfies the problem of breathing. It teaches us how to take deep breaths which purify the entire body system. There are types of breathing styles that help to clear the nasal passages and calm the nervous system. Pranayama is the best exercise for people suffering from allergies.

You can also get rid of obesity and arthritis by practicing yoga. Yoga is indeed a blessing in disguise for mankind; it is a drug that has no side effects.

Yoga – the flow of energy within us

Yoga as a way of life that is elaborate and can easily be rounded as a comprehensive workout for a person. Positive effects are further developed by yoga and had impacts on personal, psychological and spiritual well-being. Anyone who is blessed with yoga knows how yoga can have a life-changing effects on a person psyche. You will simply understand yoga as a way of life and recognize its true essence.

Yoga is definitely beyond any set of poses that improve a person's flexibility while improving posture.

Yoga encourages various physical, mental and spiritual activities. These activities help in improving a person's health standards. These are not just exercises. They are considered the source code for leading healthy lives. This is something that helps to create a link between Personal consciousness and divine consciousness.

We can all feel the greatness within us. Within Buddhism it is called Buddha nature, and within Christianity, Christ Consciousness. Call it what you want, it is there and no perfection is required on our part to make it complete.

The trouble is that not only do we see it, but we recognize that meditation, yoga, and other spiritual practices produce it. We think things like, "I will meditate to awaken my mind," as if the pure fundamental consciousness within needs awakening.

We can do this with the best of intentions, yet it is not realized that joining a meditation class or yoga studio can lead to our achievement or Spiritual ambitions. Working to become more aware and in tune with the nature of reality works under the assumptions that we are not in tune and that a certain amount of perfecting is necessary to become enlightened—or at least achieve a far greater awareness than we presently know.

Proper meditation rarely involves doing anything other than what we are doing. Are we trying to achieve something, or are we trying to achieve In our own way? A small shift in attitude can bring all the changes in the world. If we can move our thoughts from acquiring knowledge to Recognizing enlightenment, we make ourselves vulnerable to awakening and grace.

The philosophy of Yoga reminds us that the journey to master the mind is long and requires patience, practice and perseverance. Finally there is salvation from sorrow. This liberation does not involve going beyond the physical body or recognizing it. In time, with somewhere

The philosophy of yoga reminds us that the journey to mind mastery is long and requires patience, practice and perseverance. In the end there is freedom from suffering. This liberation includes going beyond or not identifying with the physical body. In time, somewhere along the journey, the yoga practitioner gets it! "I am more than the physical body!" And with this realization that she is more than the body, the liberation philosophy often proves to be a diamond worth pursuing. If the person lives mostly in her head, the goal of liberation is grasped with both hands to treasure for life. The practitioner feels validated with the glimpse of freedom.

Yoga connecting the soul of the mind

Yoga means different things to different people. Most people start yoga firstly because it can provide physical benefits. They want to lose Weight, tone up, feel healthy or perhaps help with a medical condition or physical symptoms. Yoga works on all physical conditions. There are other people who are more attracted to the emotional and / or spiritual side.

What is interesting here is that we are connected on all three levels; Mind, body and soul, so in reality when we are in a physical state that something is healing or simply being overweight or unfit, it will always be connected to our emotions and ultimately, whether we choose to believe it or No (and there are) many who do not are also connected on a subtle, spiritual level. You do not need to accept this fact to practice Yoga, but it is worth knowing that when you start that you are actually working on all three levels, *not* physical.

Breathing - a must to regulate mind

The process of controlled and proper breathing we term it as the reawakening of the inner self with which we link the energy flow of the divine.

To start with, sit in an ideal place; feel comfortable, relaxed and calmed. This place should be clean, proper ventilated with good oxygen level.
The period of sunrise is the best time to breathe. If this is not possible then follow the procedure in the evening time.

Now start breathing inhaling the breath slowly feeling inner sound. The process must be slow, very slow. The sound of breath will not be heard even by our ears, but only felt by us.

Stop for few seconds

Now exhale the breath slowly feeling inner sound. The process must be slow, very slow. The sound of breath will not be heard even by our ears, but only felt by us.

Now again stop for few seconds

Repeat the process

Do this process for 20 to 30 minutes daily.

Yes in a few weeks you will realize it's amazing effects.

Not only headache but the divine power of healing has started in the body. This will make you believe in a more positive and balanced method.

The fear of the unknown will disappear.

Proper breathing is a natural healing process. Here the deity is in the process of stopping and breathing.

Anulom Vilom Pranayama is actually very useful for our health. It is very effective for purification of the body. Anulom Antonym is an excellent breathing technique to calm and focus the mind while improving blood circulation.

Anulom Vilom Pranayama, also known as alternate nostril breathing technique, is an incredible energy, which works effectively to relieve stress and anxiety. With regular practice we can treat serious health conditions including heart problems, cartilage, depression, asthma, high blood pressure, and arthritis.

Yoga experts suggest it to be the best breathing exercise to manage stress levels, as it helps control breathing and thus, regulates the mind.

Find a Yoga teacher with mental health expertise

You can practice yoga on your own, but being with a teacher who has experience instructing people with mental health issues is especially valuable. These teachers are likely to be certified in yoga therapy, as opposed to being a more basic yoga teacher.

If you can afford some private sessions, it might be better than diving into a group class. If you are feeling anxious, for example, your teacher may modify the practice or, if you are not feeling ok, the teacher spends a lot of time sitting near you guiding.

Prana Yoga to benefit you

The power of life is known as "Prana". The word Jeeva was coined because of the existence of life in organisms. The greater the amount of life element in a creature, the more powerful, advanced and great it becomes.

At the same time, the lesser the amount of life element, the creature becomes weak, useless, lazy and low-level. The main feeling of life inside the body is considered 'Tejasvita'. Its meaning is found in the Gayatri Mantra with the word '. The word Bharg means 'fast'.

To increase the standard of living in humans, it is considered best to practice 'Pranayama'. Diet, systematic routine, relaxed and calm mind, happy mind and celibacy all work to increase the power of life in you.

The growth of vital energy in the body means to fill that wonderful element inside which human powers develop further. Through this, age can also be increased.

The effect of Pran Yoga is not limited only to our body, but its effect makes all the senses and senses within us powerful, which removes the negativity inside the mind and awakens the feeling of positivity and creativity in it. Apart from this, it also gives the seeker a feeling of happiness, and bliss. With this, the intellect of the person develops rapidly and the body is always healthy.

Desires and us

We all have desires. We are born with desires. We aspire to be happy and prosper, fulfill our dreams to love and be loved by everyone. Yes, it depends on whether you can afford them. But you still have a lot of energy. You have to be calm and simple again with this. I try to look for people for content and it is very strange.

Enjoy making other people happy; enjoying more to say that I am happy to take the students who I love to hug and I love to kiss and I love to smell and I love to feel and really feel the feeling of exchange.

I really love them; it's a commitment in love. And the most unique thing in the world in front of every one is the expression of Love and gratitude. But this is true. I grow because of that love and I need it.

You become part of the reflective energy of the group around you. And I know that when I came down for breakfast this morning and there were twenty-five people having breakfast with me and I loved them. It really made my breakfast good and I had a tough week. I saw them all and I really loved them and I felt so grateful that they came to live here with me. It is nothing that Dean has imposed on me; no one is sitting on me and making his way to my house.

It was a deep joy and deep respect and thankful to him. To be grateful to them for whatever they are, as my friends, as their children. And what are you doing until you feel like it? A living illusion. The reality is that you actually have what you want around you. Why shouldn't it happen?

It is given. Our life is given. So what is it to ask once or ask twice? Until you really feel the fact of it being given, you feel the creative flow coming through you so you understand that it is a gift, you have failed completely in asking because you haven't asked enough to get the channel open. And if the channel isn't open then you're not attached to this creative energy, you're attached to your stupidity, your tensions which don't allow you to ask enough to really get this thing moving.

I really want amazing things in my life. I want to see a change in myself every single day. And if you are able to conserve your energy, if you live in an environment that can nourish you, do not possibly build your energy to the point where it will lift you above the pattern that is bothering you. This will take you away from the volume you want to join.
You must understand, you have to be conscious in your mind, even if your feelings are not there, even if your depth is not there, you start doing the right thing because it will save your energy when you keep asking these things, you will break or surrender and you'll bring your energy in a deeper place in yourself and you'll become affected. You'll get the muscles that will support

the growth that you want

Yoga to live a long life

Yoga can have a profound and positive impact in anti-aging progress i.e. yoga for a long life, some well-known institute studies suggested.

Old age is a natural process of aging.

Ancient techniques for the harmony of the outer and inner body beings through yoga, breath control, meditation, physical movement and gestures well known to the people of the Western world and parts of Asia.There are reasons for the reported health benefits by reputable institutions.

Researchers, in a study of yoga breathing in the skin protected against aging, reported the following results

1. Yoga breathing has reduced the psychological aspects of stress and anxiety that have been associated with increasing age. Yoga breathing (Pranayama) can have a significant and positive effect in bringing the mind to the present moment and reducing stress

2. Yoga also affected regulated glycation and products (AGE), which have recently been shown to play a role in aging

3. Comprehensive yoga programs that include inhalation and meditation exercises may have profound effects in increased gene expression, including oxidative stress, DNA damage, cell cycle control, aging, and apoptosis.

4. Yoga delayed the aging process through the expression of victims of breathing depression, anxiety, traumatic stress disorder, and mass disasters.

5 Sadhana relieve many kinds of suffering.

Finally, after taking other risk factors into consideration, researchers concluded that yoga breathing may affect the longevity mechanism.

Yoga does great for body and soul, especially for more than 60 of us. Here are some examples of vibrant women whose devotion to yoga has paid off in happiness, health and longevity:

So how does it work? How, in particular, does yoga benefit your body and mind?

In terms of your body, yoga improves balance, which continues to increase as we age. Yoga promotes bone strength, as the nature of the movements themselves improves bone density, which decreases over time. Yoga is a low-impact form of exercise, which means it gently strengthens your muscles, and in the process, protects them from atrophying. Stronger muscles mean less stress on your joints, thus reducing arthritis.

Yoga also reduces blood pressure without putting undue pressure on your cardiovascular system, which is why it is (for most people, always check with your doctor!) Particularly favorable as part of a low blood pressure-blood pressure program. Because yoga incorporates deep breathing as a part of practice, more oxygen is circulated throughout the body, for the benefit of your entire internal organs and systems.

Plus side to your mental and emotional state, yoga stimulates some chemical release in the body which can reduce anxiety and promote an overall feeling of relaxation. Because yoga relieves stress, many people find that it improves their sleep. With that said, yoga has been shown to enhance your memory and ability to process cognitively, something we can all appreciate as we grow in later years!

Why is it important to know about the benefits of yoga? Because it lends itself to a little-known health trick: the more you know how much a thing benefits you, the greater the benefit.

Harness the power of your mind by engaging in the practice of yoga. Know the value and benefits that yoga has for you, both physically and mentally. You can't help but thrive!

Taken as a whole, yoga may have a therapeutic effect in the progression of aging through regulating cellular and psychological manifestations alone or combined with meditation.

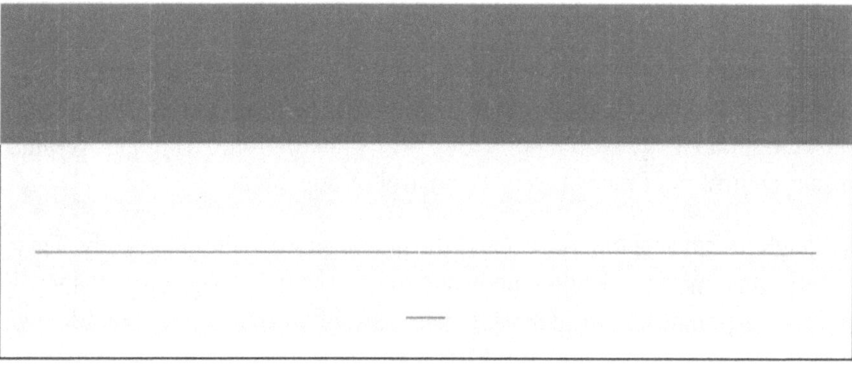

Yoga journey for everyone

Yoga as a way of life that is elaborate and can easily roundup as a comprehensive workout for a person. Yoga develops positive effects and have an impact on personal, psychological, and spiritual well-being. For anyone who is blessed with yoga, knows deeply how yoga art can have life-changing effects for one's psyche. You will just come to understand yoga as a way of life and recognize its true essence.

Yoga is definitely beyond any set of poses that improve a person's flexibility while improving posture.

Yoga correlates various physical, mental and spiritual activities. These activities help in improving a person's health standards. These are not just exercises. They are considered to be the source code for leading a healthy life. This is something that helps to create a link between individual consciousness and divine consciousness.

What is the benefit of doing this? This asana is very effective in improving overall lung capacity. Taking the air in and leaving at full strength will help remove carbon residue from the body. In addition, a surplus supply of oxygen helps in purification of blood. Performing this asana regularly will help in healing the lungs

Let us consider **Ashtanga** yoga for an example. Ashtanga yoga is an ancient practice that focuses on cleansing and purifying the body. This is achieved by synchronized body breath and movement. Ashtanga yoga tones the nervous system and also inspires spiritual enlightenment over time.

Pranayama: a way to achieve higher states of awareness. A very interesting word related to yoga is pranayama. Let us know more about the same. Prana refers to vital energy within our body. This is the life force within us. Ayama means control. So Pranayama is the control of breathing.

Through pranayama one can control the pranic energy within the body. This ensures that one has a healthy body and mind. The great yoga guru, Patanjali, referred to pranayama to achieve higher states of awareness. First of all, yoga is a great option for inner peace. With pranayams one can feel inner peace which essentially translates to breathing technique and control. Regulation of air in our body increases metabolism in our system as well as oxygen, which keeps us fresh and energetic.

Kapalabhati: An implementation of Pranayama. Kapalabhati is a yoga technique and a type of pranayama. It initially sounds like a breathing technique, but in short, Kapalbhati has a deeper meaning.

Kapalbhati is a cleansing technique that clears the mind of carbon dioxide. Kapalbhati also clears the mind of restlessness.

The technique was invented thousands of years ago by Indian yogis. It is believed to be a way of achieving full body fitness. Numerous patients have benefitted greatly by making Kapalbhati a part of their everyday lives.

Benefits of Surya Namaskar

Let us discuss another important word related to yoga, which is Surya Namaskar or Surya Namaskar. Surya Namaskar is an activity performed in the morning at sunrise. It is a compilation of twelve lines, with each pose flowing smoothly to the next section.

Surya Namaskar can be done at a fast pace, or it can be done slowly. A unique feature of Surya Namaskar is that it is a complete workout for the body. While it consists of only 12 sets of exercises, Surya Namaskar has become 288 powerful yoga poses. It occurs over a period of 12 to 15 minutes.

In one round, Surya Namaskar burns around 13.90 calories. Slowly and slowly, you can increase the rounds of Surya Namaskar to 108.

If performed at a slow pace, Surya Namaskar tones the muscles and makes them stronger. Alternatively, Surya Namaskar brings the mind, body and breath in harmony and facilitates a complete meditation experience.

If one performs only a few rounds of Surya Namaskar, it can be very good for the heart. If you want to do Surya Namaskar as a hot workout, you can do it at a fast pace.

More benefits of yoga

• Then there are several poses to try. They aim to increase your flexibility and balance.

• They also target core muscles and make them stronger.

• Yoga is also very good for weight loss and pain relief.

• Since it moves slowly, there is not much stress on the body to perform and maintain.

• One can do them at a steady pace and aim for perfection of each pose for best results.

• If you are highly ambitious and have a fit body that is used to working, you can try Surya Namaskar. It is a combination of 10 poses, with alternate breathing and breathing patterns for each pose. Needless to say, it targets every part of your body and it can be effective.

Yoga as a way of life is a very wide field and is not limited to physical activities only. There are many meditation poses that help bring the right balance in your life. Due to stress and anxiety, there are examples of which a person is suffering from various diseases due to these. To deal with these problems, you need to do yoga asanas.

Lotus posture is very effective for dealing with stress and anxiety. In this, the practitioner needs to sit with bent legs and has to breathe vigorously. It helps in improving the blood flow in the body and relieving stress.

As you build proximity to nature, you come to know that it is natural resources that hold the key to eternal health and well-being and making yoga as a way of life.